The Complete Mediterra
Cookbook for Beginr

MW00508320

Quick & Easy Delicious Recipes - Change your
Eating Lifestyle with 4-Week Meal Plan!

Kenneth Anderson

Table of Contents

BREAKFAST

01. Raspberries and Yogurt Smoothie

Preparation time: 5 minutes

Cooking time: 0 minutes

Servings:2

- Ingredients:
- 2 cups raspberries
- ½ cup Greek yogurt
- ½ cup almond milk
- ½ teaspoon vanilla extract

Directions:

1. In your blender, combine the raspberries with the milk, vanilla and the yogurt, pulse well, divide into 2 glasses and serve for breakfast.

Nutrition Values:calories 245, fat 9.5, fiber 2.3, carbs 5.6, protein 1.6

02. Farro Salad

Preparation time: 5 minutes

Cooking time: 4 minutes

Servings:2

Ingredients:

- 1 tablespoon olive oil
- A pinch of salt and black pepper
- 1 bunch baby spinach, chopped
- 1 avocado, pitted, peeled and chopped
- 1 garlic clove, minced
- 2 cups farro, already cooked
- ½ cup cherry tomatoes, cubed

Directions:

1. Heat up a pan with the oil over medium heat, add the spinach, and the rest of the ingredients, toss, cook for 4 minutes, divide into bowls and serve.

Nutrition Values:calories 157, fat 13.7, fiber 5.5, carbs 8.6, protein 3.6

03. Cranberry and Dates Squares

Preparation time: 30 minutes

Cooking time: 0 minutes

Servings:10

Ingredients:

- 12 dates, pitted and chopped
- 1 teaspoon vanilla extract
- ¼ cup honey
- ½ cup rolled oats
- ¾ cup cranberries, dried
- ¼ cup almond avocado oil, melted
- 1 cup walnuts, roasted and chopped
- ¼ cup pumpkin seeds

Directions:

2. In a bowl, mix the dates with the vanilla, honey and the rest of the ingredients, stir well and press everything on a baking sheet lined with parchment paper.
3. Keep in the freezer for 30 minutes, cut into 10 squares and serve for breakfast.

Nutrition Values:calories 263, fat 13.4, fiber 4.7, carbs 14.3. protein 3.5

04. Cheesy Eggs Ramekins

Preparation time: 10 minutes

Cooking time: 10 minutes

Servings:2

Ingredients:

- 1 tablespoon chives, chopped
- 1 tablespoon dill, chopped
- A pinch of salt and black pepper
- 2 tablespoons cheddar cheese, grated

- 1 tomato, chopped

- 2 eggs, whisked

- Cooking spray

Directions:

1. In a bowl, mix the eggs with the tomato and the rest of the ingredients except the cooking spray and whisk well.

2. Grease 2 ramekins with the cooking spray, divide the mix into each ramekin, bake at 400 degrees F for 10 minutes and serve.

Nutrition Values:calories 104, fat 7.1, fiber 0.6, carbs 2.6, protein 7.9

SEAFOOD

05. Baked Trout and Fennel

Preparation time: 10 minutes

Cooking time: 22 minutes

Servings:4

Ingredients:

- fennel bulb, sliced

- tablespoons olive oil

- yellow onion, sliced

- teaspoons Italian seasoning

- rainbow trout fillets, boneless

- ¼ cup panko breadcrumbs

- ½ cup kalamata olives, pitted and halved

- Juice of 1 lemon

Directions:

1. Spread the fennel the onion and the rest of the ingredients except the trout and the breadcrumbs on a baking sheet lined with parchment paper, toss them and cook at 400 degrees F for 10 minutes.

2. Add the fish dredged in breadcrumbs and seasoned with salt and pepper and cook it at 400 degrees F for 6 minutes on each side.

3. Divide the mix between plates and serve.

Nutrition Values:calories 306, fat 8.9, fiber 11.1, carbs 23.8, protein 14.5

06. Lemon Rainbow Trout

Preparation time: 10 minutes

Cooking time: 15 minutes

Servings:2

Ingredients:

- rainbow trout
- Juice of 1 lemon
- tablespoons olive oil
- garlic cloves, minced
- A pinch of salt and black pepper

Directions:

1. Line a baking sheet with parchment paper, add the fish and the rest of the ingredients and rub.
2. Bake at 400 degrees F for 15 minutes, divide between plates and serve with a side salad.

Nutrition Values:calories 521, fat 29, fiber 5, carbs 14, protein 52

07. Trout and Peppers Mix

Preparation time: 10 minutes

Cooking time: 20 minutes

Servings:4

Ingredients:

- trout fillets, boneless

- tablespoons kalamata olives, pitted and chopped
- tablespoon capers, drained
- tablespoons olive oil
- A pinch of salt and black pepper
- and ½ teaspoons chili powder
- yellow bell pepper, chopped
- red bell pepper, chopped
- green bell pepper, chopped

Directions:

1. Heat up a pan with the oil over medium-high heat, add the trout, salt and pepper and cook for 10 minutes.
2. Flip the fish, add the peppers and the rest of the ingredients, cook for 10 minutes more, divide the whole mix between plates and serve.

Nutrition Values:calories 572, fat 17.4, fiber 6, carbs 71, protein 33.7

08. Cod and Cabbage

Preparation time: 10 minutes

Cooking time: 15 minutes

Servings:4

Ingredients:

- cups green cabbage, shredded
- sweet onion, sliced
- A pinch of salt and black pepper
- ½ cup feta cheese, crumbled
- teaspoons olive oil
- 4 cod fillets, boneless
- ¼ cup green olives, pitted and chopped

Directions:

1. Grease a roasting pan with the oil, add the fish, the cabbage and the rest of the ingredients, introduce in the pan and cook at 450 degrees F for 15 minutes.
2. Divide the mix between plates and serve.

Nutrition Values:calories 270, fat 10, fiber 3, carbs 12, protein 31

09. Mediterranean Mussels

Preparation time: 10 minutes

Cooking time: 10 minutes

Servings:4

Ingredients:

- white onion, sliced
- tablespoons olive oil
- teaspoons fennel seeds
- garlic cloves, minced
- teaspoon red pepper, crushed
- A pinch of salt and black pepper
- cup chicken stock
- tablespoon lemon juice
- and ½ pounds mussels, scrubbed
- ½ cup parsley, chopped
- ½ cup tomatoes, cubed

Directions:

1. Heat up a pan with the oil over medium-high heat, add the onion and the garlic and sauté for 2 minutes.
2. Add the rest of the ingredients except the mussels, stir and cook for 3 minutes more.
3. Add the mussels, cook everything for 6 minutes more, divide everything into bowls and serve.

10. Mussels Bowls

Preparation time: 10 minutes

Cooking time: 10 minutes

Servings:4

Ingredients:

- 2 pounds mussels, scrubbed
- tablespoon garlic, minced
- tablespoon basil, chopped
- yellow onion, chopped
- tomatoes, cubed
- cup heavy cream
- tablespoons olive oil
- tablespoon parsley, chopped

Directions:

1. Heat up a pan with the oil over medium-high heat, add the garlic and the onion and sauté for 2 minutes.
2. Add the mussels and the rest of the ingredients, toss, cook for 7 minutes more, divide into bowls and serve.

Nutrition Values:calories 266, fat 11.8, fiber 5.8, carbs 16.5, protein 10.5

POULTRY

11. Amazing Chicken Salad

Preparation time: 30 minutes

Cooking time: 20 minutes

Servings:4

Ingredients:

- 4 medium chicken breasts, boneless and skinless
- 2 eggplants, sliced
- Salt and black pepper to taste
- tablespoon ginger, grated
- tablespoon garlic, minced
- tablespoons balsamic vinegar
- tablespoons olive oil
- tablespoons red wine
- ¼ teaspoon chili paste

For the vinaigrette:

- teaspoon ginger, grated

- teaspoons balsamic vinegar

- teaspoons Dijon mustard

- teaspoon brown sugar

- tablespoons olive oil

- tablespoon lime juice

For serving:

- ½ lettuce head, leaves torn

- pound cucumbers, sliced

- ¾ cup cilantro, chopped

- ½ cup scallions, sliced

- red chili pepper, chopped

Directions:

1. In a bowl, mix 1 tablespoon grated ginger with 1 tablespoon minced garlic, 2 tablespoons balsamic vinegar, 3 tablespoons olive oil, 2 tablespoon red wine and ½ teaspoon chili paste.

2. Whisk well. Place eggplant slices in a bowl, add half of the marinade and toss to coat.

3. Place chicken breasts in another bowl, add the rest of the ginger marinade. Toss to coat and set aside for 30 minutes.

4. Heat up a kitchen grill over medium high heat, add eggplant slices, cook for 3 minutes on each side and transfer them to a bowl. Arrange chicken breasts on grill, cook for 5 minutes, flip and cook for 2 more minutes, transfer them to a cutting board, leave aside for 4 minutes and then slice them.

5. Arrange lettuce leaves on a platter, add chicken slices, grilled eggplant slices, cucumbers and scallions and some salt.

6. In a bowl, mix 2 teaspoons balsamic vinegar with 1 teaspoon grated ginger, brown sugar, mustard, 3 tablespoons olive oil, salt to the taste and lime juice and stir well.

7. Spread 1 tablespoon of this vinaigrette over eggplant and chicken salad. Add cilantro, chopped chili on top and serve.

Nutrition Values:calories 264, fat 14, fiber 6, carbs 8, protein 5

12. Delicious Chicken Soup

Preparation time: 10 minutes

Cooking time: 1 hour

Servings:8

Ingredients:

- 2 cups eggplant, diced
- Salt and black pepper to taste
- ¼ cup olive oil + 1 tablespoon
- cup yellow onion, chopped
- tablespoons garlic, minced
- red bell pepper, chopped
- tablespoons hot paprika+ 2 teaspoons
- ¼ cup parsley, chopped
- teaspoon turmeric
- and ½ tablespoons oregano, chopped
- cups chicken stock
- pound chicken breast, skinless, boneless and cut into small pieces
- cup half and half
- and ½ tablespoons cornstarch
- egg yolks
- ¼ cup lemon juice
- Lemon wedges for serving

Directions:

1. In a bowl, mix eggplant pieces with ¼ cup oil, salt and pepper to taste and toss to coat.

2. Arrange eggplant on a lined baking sheet, place in the oven at 400 degrees F and bake for 10 minutes.

3. Flip, cook for 10 minutes more and set aside to cool.

4. Heat a saucepan with 1 tablespoon oil over medium heat, add garlic and onion, cover and cook for 10 minutes.

5. Add bell pepper, stir and cook uncovered for 3 minutes.

6. Add hot paprika, ginger and turmeric and stir well.

7. Add the stock, chicken, eggplant pieces, oregano and parsley.

8. Stir, bring to a boil and simmer for 12 minutes.

9. In a bowl, mix cornstarch with half and half and egg yolks - stir well.

10. Add 1 cup soup, stir again and pour gradually into soup.

11. Stir, add salt and pepper to taste and lemon juice. Ladle into soup bowls and serve with lemon wedges on the side.

Nutrition Values:calories 242, fat 3, fiber 2, carbs 5, protein 3

13. Mediterranean Chicken and Lentil Soup

Preparation time: 10 minutes

Cooking time: 1 hour and 10 minutes

Servings:8

Ingredients:

- 4 tablespoons butter
- 2 celery stalks, chopped

- 2 carrots, chopped
- yellow onion, chopped
- tablespoons tomato paste
- garlic cloves, chopped
- cups chicken stock
- 2 cups French lentils
- pound chicken thighs, skinless and boneless
- Salt and black pepper to taste
- Grated parmesan for serving

Directions:

1. Heat a Dutch oven with the butter over medium high heat, add onion, garlic, carrots and celery, stir and cook for 6 minutes.
2. Add salt and pepper to taste, stir and cook for 4 more minutes.
3. Add tomato paste, stir and cook for 2 minutes. Add lentils, chicken stock and chicken thighs, stir, bring to a boil, cover oven and cook for 1 hour.
4. Transfer chicken thighs to a plate and leave aside to cool down.
5. Transfer soup to a food processor, add more salt and pepper if needed and blend.
6. Return soup to oven, shred chicken meat and add to oven.
7. Stir, ladle into soup bowls, sprinkle cheese on top and serve.

Nutrition Values:calories 231, fat 2, fiber 2, carbs 5, protein 3

14. Classic Mediterranean Chicken Soup

Preparation time: 15 minutes

Cooking time: 1 hour and 20 minutes

Servings:4

Ingredients:

- big chicken
- tablespoons salt
- cups water
- leek, cut in quarters
- bay leaves
- carrot, cut into quarters
- tablespoons olive oil
- 2/3 cup rice
- cups yellow onion, chopped
- eggs
- ½ cup lemon juice
- teaspoon black pepper

Directions:

1. Put chicken in a large saucepan, add water and 2 tablespoons salt, bring to a boil over medium high heat, reduce heat and skim foam.

2. Add carrot, bay leaves and leek and simmer for 1 hour.

3. Heat a pan with the oil over medium high heat, add onion, stir and cook for 6

minutes, take off heat and leave aside for now.

4. Transfer chicken to a cutting board and leave aside to cool down.

5. Strain soup back into the saucepan.

6. Add sautéed onion and rice, bring again to a boil over high heat, reduce temperature to low and simmer for 20 minutes.

7. Discard chicken bones and skin, dice into big chunks and return to boiling soup.

8. Meanwhile, in a bowl, mix lemon juice with eggs and black pepper and stir well.

9. Add 2 cups boiling soup and whisk again well.

10. Pour this into the soup and stir well.

11. Add remaining salt, stir, take off heat, transfer to soup bowls and serve right away.

Nutrition Values:calories 242, fat 3, fiber 2, carbs 3, protein 3

15. Delicious Chicken Sausage and Peppers

Servings: 6

Preparationtime: 10 minutes Cook time: 20 minutes

Ingredients:

- Green pepper finely cut
- 1 onion finely cut
- 1 red pepper seeded and cut
- 1/2 cup dry white wine
- 1/2 teaspoon sea salt
- 1/4 teaspoon black pepper
- tablespoons olive oil
- garlic cloves minced
- Italian chicken sausage
- Red pepper flakes

Directions:

1. In a vast skillet over medium-high heat heat the olive oil until it simmers.
2. add the sausages and cook for 5 to 7 minutes until browned and they achieve an internal temperature of 165°F. With help of tongs expel the sausage from the skillet and put aside on a platter tented with aluminum foil to keep warm.
3. Back to the skillet to add the onion red pepper and green pepper. Cook for 5 to 7

minutes mixing them until the vegetables start to browned.

4. add the garlic and cook for 30 seconds,

5. mix in the wine sea salt pepper and red pepper pieces. Use the side of a spoon to rub and overlap in any browned bits from the base of the pan. Stew for around 4 minutes blend until the fluid reduces considerably. Spoon the peppers over the sausage and serve.

16. Tasty Chicken Piccata

Servings: 6

Preparationtime: 10 minutes

Cooking time: 15 minutes

Ingredients:

- tablespoons virgin olive oil
- 1 glass unsalted chicken broth
- Juice of 1 lemon
- Zest of 1 lemon
- 1/2 glass wheat flour
- 1/2 teaspoon sea salt
- 1/2 pounds boneless skinless chicken breast cut into 6 pieces and pounded V2-inch thick (see tip)
- 1/2. glass dry white wine
- 1/4 glass capers rinsed
- 1/4 glass chopped parsley leaves
- 1/8 teaspoon black pepper

Directions:

1. In a little bowl mix the flour sea salt and pepper. Dig the chicken in the flour and tap off any excess..
2. In a vast pan over medium-high heat heat the olive oil until it simmers.
3. add the chicken and cook for around 4 minutes for every side until browned. Expel

the chicken from the skillet and put aside overlap with aluminum foil to keep warm.

4. Back to the the skillet to the heat and mix the wine lemon juice and lemon zest. Use the side of a spoon to rub and overlap in any browned bits from the base of the pan. Stew for 3 to 4 minutes mixing until the fluid thickens. Expel the skillet from the heat and put the chicken to the dish. Swing to coat. Blend in the parsley and serve. Between two bits of cling wrap or material paper and use a level kitchen hammer or a smooth-bottomed overwhelming pan to pound until they achieve the ideal thickness. Use caution to avoid from puncturing the plastic or paper.

17. One-Pan Delectable Tuscan Chicken

Servings: 6

Preparationtime: 10 minutes

Cooking time: 25 minutes

Ingredients:

- 1 (14-ounce) cup sliced tomatoes.

- 1 (14-ounce) cup crushed tomatoes

- 1 (14-ounce) cup white beans

- 1 onion sliced

- 1 pound boneless skinless chicken breast cut into 34-inch pieces

- 1 red pepper.

- 1 tablespoon dried Italian seasoning

- 1/2 teaspoon sea salt

- 1/4 cup basil leaves

- 1/4 cup olive oil.

- 1/8 teaspoon black pepper

- 1/8 teaspoon red pepper flakes

- 3 garlic cloves minced

Directions:

1. 1.In a vast pan over medium heat heat 2 tablespoons of olive oil until it simmers.

2. 2.Add the chicken and cook for around 6 minutes mixing until browned. Expel the chicken from the skillet and put aside on a platter overlap with aluminum foil to

keep warm.

3. 3.Back to the skillet and heat the rest of the 2 tablespoons of olive oil until it simmers

4. 4.combine the onion and red pepper. Cook for around 5 minutes until the vegetables are delicate.

5. 5.add the garlic and cook for 30 seconds.

6. 6.whisk in the wine and use the side of the spoon to rub and overlap in any seared bits from the base of the dish. Cook for 1 minute.

7. 7.mix crushed tomatoes white beans. Italian flavoring sea salt pepper and red pepper flakes. Take a stew and decrease the heat to medium. Cook for 5 minutes.

8. 8.back to the chicken and any juices that have gathered to the skillet. Cook for 1 to 2 minutes until the chicken warms through. Expel from the heat and mix in the basil before serving.

MAIN DISH

18. Creamy Chicken Soup

Preparation time: 10 minutes

Cooking time: 1 hour

Servings:8

Ingredients:

- 2 cups eggplant, cubed

- Salt and black pepper to the taste

- ¼ cup olive oil

- 1 yellow onion, chopped

- 2 tablespoons garlic, minced

- 1 red bell pepper, chopped

- 2 tablespoons hot paprika

- ¼ cup parsley, chopped

- 1 and ½ tablespoons oregano, chopped

- 4 cups chicken stock

- 1 pound chicken breast, skinless, boneless and cubed

- 1 cup half and half

- 2 egg yolks

- ¼ cup lime juice

Directions:

1. Heat up a pot with the oil over medium heat, add the chicken, garlic and onion, and brown for 10 minutes.
2. Add the bell pepper and the rest of the ingredients except the half and half, egg, yolks and the lime juice, bring to a simmer and cook over medium heat for 40 minutes.
3. In a bowl, combine the egg yolks with the remaining ingredients with 1 cup of soup, whisk well and pour into the pot.
4. Whisk the soup, cook for 5 minutes more, divide into bowls and serve.

Nutrition Values:calories 312, fat 17.4, fiber 5.6, carbs 20.2, protein 15.3

19. Chicken, Carrots and Lentils Soup

Preparation time: 10 minutes

Cooking time: 1 hour and 10 minutes

Servings:8

Ingredients:

- 4 tablespoons olive oil
- 2 carrots, chopped
- 1 yellow onion, chopped
- 2 tablespoons tomato paste
- 2 garlic cloves, chopped
- 6 cups chicken stock
- 2 cups brown lentils, dried
- 1 pound chicken thighs, skinless, boneless and cubed
- Salt and black pepper to the taste

Directions:

1. Heat up a pot with the oil over medium high heat, add the chicken, onion and the garlic and brown for 10 minutes.
2. Add the rest of the ingredients, bring the soup to a boil and simmer for 1 hour.
3. Ladle the soup into bowls and serve for lunch.

Nutrition Values:calories 311, fat 13.2, fiber 4.3, carbs 17.5, protein 13.4

20. Pork and Rice Soup

Preparation time: 5 minutes

Cooking time: 7 hours

Servings:4

Ingredients:

- 2 pounds pork stew meat, cubed
- A pinch of salt and black pepper
- 6 cups water
- 1 leek, sliced
- 2 bay leaves
- 1 carrot, sliced
- 3 tablespoons olive oil
- 1 cup white rice
- 2 cups yellow onion, chopped
- ½ cup lemon juice
- 1 tablespoon cilantro, chopped

Directions:

1. In your slow cooker, combine the pork with the water and the rest of the ingredients except the cilantro, put the lid on and cook on Low for 7 hours.
2. Stir the soup, ladle into bowls, sprinkle the cilantro on top and serve.

Nutrition Values:calories 300, fat 15, fiber 7.6, carbs 17.4, protein 22.4

21. Barley and Chicken Soup

Preparation time: 10 minutes

Cooking time: 50 minutes

Servings:6

Ingredients:

- 1 pound chicken breasts, skinless, boneless and cubed
- 1 tablespoon olive oil
- Salt and black pepper to the taste
- 2 celery stalks, chopped
- 2 carrots, chopped
- 1 red onion, chopped
- 6 cups chicken stock
- ½ cup parsley, chopped
- ½ cup barley
- 1 teaspoon lime juice

Directions:

1. Heat up a pot with the oil over medium high heat, add the chicken, season with salt and pepper, and brown for cook for 8 minutes.
2. Add the onion, carrots and the celery, stir and cook for 3 minutes more.
3. Add the rest of the ingredients except the parsley, bring to a boil and simmer over medium heat for 40 minutes.
4. Add the parsley, stir, divide the soup into bowls and serve.

22. Mushrooms and Chicken Soup

Preparation time: 10 minutes

Cooking time: 30 minutes

Servings:4

Ingredients:

- 1 red onion, chopped
- 1 tablespoon olive oil
- 2 celery stalks, chopped
- 2 garlic cloves, minced
- 2 carrots chopped
- Salt and black pepper to the taste
- 1 tablespoon thyme, chopped
- 1 qt chicken stock
- 4 ounces white mushrooms, sliced
- 1 cup heavy cream
- 4 cups rotisserie chicken, shredded
- 2 tablespoons cilantro, chopped

Directions:

1. Heat up a pot with the oil over medium heat, add the onion, celery, garlic, carrot and thyme, and sauté for 5 minutes.
2. Add the rest of the ingredients except the cream and the cilantro, stir, bring to a boil and cook for 20 minutes.

3. Add the cream and cilantro, stir, cook the soup for 5 minutes more, divide everything into bowls and serve.

Nutrition Values: calories 287, fat 11.3, fiber 8.7, carbs 22.4, protein 14.4

23. Pork and Lentils Soup

Preparation time: 10 minutes

Cooking time: 1 hour

Servings:6

Ingredients:

- 1 yellow onion, chopped
- 1 tablespoon olive oil
- 2 teaspoons basil, dried
- 1 and ½ teaspoons ginger, grated
- 3 garlic cloves, chopped
- Salt and black pepper to the taste
- 1 carrot, chopped
- 1 pound pork stew meat, cubed
- 3 ounces brown lentils, rinsed
- 4 cups chicken stock
- 2 tablespoons tomato paste
- 2 tablespoons lime juice

Directions:

1. Heat up a pot with the oil over medium heat, add the meat, onion and the garlic and brown for 6 minutes.
2. Add the rest of the ingredients, bring the soup to a boil and cook for 55 minutes.
3. Divide the soup into bowls and serve.

Nutrition Values:calories 263, fat 11.3, fiber 4.5, carbs 24.4, protein 14.4

SIDE DISH

24. Beet And Cheese Side Salad

Preparation time: 15 minutes

Cooking time: 0 minutes

Servings: 6

Ingredients:

- 2 pounds beets, baked, peeled and cubed

- 2 tablespoons olive oil

- 1 tablespoon lemon juice

- 2 tablespoons red wine vinegar

- 1 cup blue cheese, crumbled

- 3 small garlic cloves, minced

- 4 green onions, chopped

- 5 tablespoons dill, chopped

- Salt and black pepper to taste

Directions:

1. In a bowl, mix vinegar with oil, lemon juice, garlic, salt and pepper, whisk well and leave aside.
2. Add green onions, cheese, beets and dill and toss to coat.

3. Leave in the fridge for 15 minutes and then serve as a side dish.

Nutrition : calories 180, fat 2, fiber 3, carbs 2, protein 3

25. Broccoli Side Dish

Preparation time: 10 minutes

Cooking time: 30 minutes

Servings:5

Ingredients:

- 2 and ½ cups quinoa
- 4 and ½ cups veggie stock
- ½ teaspoon salt
- 2 tablespoons pesto sauce
- 2 tablespoons arrowroot powder
- 12 ounces mozzarella cheese
- 2 cups spinach
- 12 ounces broccoli
- 1/3 cup parmesan
- 3 green onions, chopped

Directions:

1. Put quinoa and green onions in a baking dish.
2. Put broccoli in a heatproof bowl, place in the microwave, cook on high for 5 minutes and leave a side.
3. In a bowl, mix veggie stock with arrowroot powder, pesto sauce and some salt, stir well, transfer to a saucepan and bring to a boil over medium heat.
4. Pour over quinoa, add broccoli, spinach, parmesan and mozzarella cheese.

5. Place in the oven at 400 degrees F and bake for 30 minutes. Divide between plates and serve.

Nutrition Values:calories 210, fat 2, fiber 2, carbs 3, protein 3

26. Spicy Pea Salad

Preparation time: 10 minutes

Cooking time: 0 minutes

Servings:8

Ingredients:

- 60 ounces peas
- 1 yellow bell pepper, chopped
- 2 ounces Cheddar cheese, grated
- ½ cup mayonnaise
- 3 tablespoon basil, dried
- 2 tablespoons red onion, chopped
- 2 teaspoons chili pepper, chopped
- 1 teaspoon apple cider vinegar
- 1 teaspoon sugar
- Salt and black pepper to taste
- 1 teaspoon garlic powder
- A drizzle of hot sauce

Directions:

1. In a salad bowl, mix bell pepper with cheese, onion, basil, chili pepper, salt and pepper and stir.
2. Add mayo, sugar, vinegar, hot sauce and garlic powder and stir.
3. Add peas, toss well, place in the fridge and serve cold as a side dish.

Nutritional value: calories 120, fat 2, fiber 1, carbs 2, protein 3

27. Mashed Potatoes

Preparation time: 10 minutes

Cooking time: 40 minutes

Servings:10

Ingredients:

- 2 pounds gold potatoes, cut into small pieces
- 1 ½ cup fresh ricotta cheese
- Sea salt and black pepper to taste
- ½ cup low fat milk
- 3 tablespoons butter

Directions:

1. Put potatoes in a large saucepan, add water to cover, add a pinch of salt, bring to a simmer over medium heat, cook for 20 minutes then drain and mash well.
2. Add salt, pepper, milk, butter and ricotta and stir well.
3. Spoon mashed potatoes into 10 ramekins, place in a baking pan and broil them for a few minutes. Serve hot.

Nutrition Values: calories 180, fat 3, fiber 1, carbs 2, protein 3

28. Brown Rice and Tomatoes

Preparation time: 5 minutes

Cooking time: 50 minutes

Servings:4

Ingredients:

- 1 tablespoon olive oil
- 1 cup brown rice
- 1 yellow onion, chopped
- 1 tablespoon tomato paste
- 2 tomatoes, cubed
- A pinch of salt and black pepper
- 1 tablespoon basil, chopped
- 2 cups hot water

Directions:

1. Heat a pan with the oil over medium high heat.
2. Add the onion, tomatoes, salt, pepper and the tomato paste, stir and cook for 5 minutes.
3. Add the rice and the water, stir, bring to a simmer and cook over medium heat for 45 minutes.
4. Add the basil, toss, divide the mix between plates and serve as a side dish.

Nutrition Values: calories 187, fat 7, fiber 4, carbs 7, protein 3

29. Creamy Barley Side Salad

Preparation time: 15 minutes

Cooking time: 30 minutes

Servings:4

Ingredients:

- ½ cup barley
- 1 and ½ cup water
- ½ cup Greek yogurt
- Salt and black pepper to taste
- 2 tablespoons olive oil
- 1 teaspoon mustard
- 1 tablespoon lemon juice
- 2 celery stalks, sliced
- ¼ cup mint, chopped
- 1 apple, cored and chopped

Directions:

1. Put barley in a pan, add water and some salt, bring to a boil, cover, simmer for 25 minutes, drain, arrange on a baking sheet and leave aside.
2. In a bowl, mix yogurt with lemon juice, oil, salt, pepper and mustard and stir well.
3. Add mint, apple, celery and barley, toss to coat and serve.

Nutrition Values:calories 132, fat 2, fiber 3, carbs 3, protein 1

SOUPS AND STEWS

For more tips go to: Growthshape.com/health

30. Special Delicious Veggie Soup

Preparation time:1 hour

Servings: 8

Ingredients:

- Cored and diced yellow bell pepper - 1

- Sliced celery stalk – 1

- Chopped garlic clove - 1

- Chopped sweet onion – 1

- Peeled and cubed pounds potatoes – 1 ½

- Vegetable stock – 2 cups

- Water – 7 cups

- Olive oil – 2 tbsps.

- Greek yogurt for serving – ½ cup

- Pepper and salt to taste

- Diced carrots - 2

Directions:

- Stir in a soup pot carrots, onion, pepper, celery, garlic and heated oil.

- Add salt, potatoes, water, pepper and stock after cooking for 5 minutes.

- On low heat, cook the soup for 20 minutes.

- Remove from heat when the soup is done. Then pour it into serving bowls.

- Add Greek yogurt when serving.

31. Sweet Onion Soup

Servings 6

Preparation Time: 40 minutes

Ingredients:

- Olive oil - 4 tbsp.
- Rosemary - 1 sprig
- Sweet onions - 4, sliced
- Thyme - 1 sprig
- Vegetable stock - 3 cups
- Water - 2 cups
- Gruyere cheese – 4 oz., grated
- Dry white wine - ¼ cup
- Salt and pepper - to taste

Directions:

1. Put olive oil into a pot and heat, adding in the onions and stir. Cook onions until caramelized, which should take about 15 minutes.
2. Pour in water, vegetable stock, wine, rosemary and thyme. Season with salt and pepper to suit your taste.
3. Soup should cook on low for about 15 minutes and then it is complete.
4. Sprinkle cheese on top and eat while hot.

32. Very Veggie Soup

Servings 8

Preparation Time: 1 hour

Ingredients:

- Olive oil - 2 tbsp.

- Stalk of celery - 1, sliced

- Garlic clove - 1, chopped

- Sweet onion - 1, chopped

- Small fennel bulb - 1, sliced

- Carrot - 1, diced

- Potatoes - 2, peeled and cubed

- Leek - 1, sliced

- Tomatoes - 2, peeled and diced

- Chicken stock - 4 cups

- Water - 4 cups

- Tomato paste - 2 tbsp.

- Salt and pepper - to taste

Directions:

1. Pour olive oil into a pot and heat. Add in celery, garlic, onion, fennel, carrot and leek, stirring well.

2. After cooking for 5 minutes you can stir in water, chicken stock and potatoes. Add salt and pepper to suit your personal taste.

3. Set heat to low and cook for 25 minutes.

4. Soup is hot and ready to eat.

33. Delicious Bean Soup

Preparation time: 10 minutes

Cooking time: 1 hour

Servings:4

Ingredients:

- 1 tomato, chopped

- 1 garlic clove, minced

- cups fava beans, dried

- cups water

- 1 small yellow onion, chopped

- 1 tablespoon olive oil

- Salt and black pepper to taste

- ¼ teaspoon cumin, ground

- ¼ teaspoon saffron threads, crushed

Directions:

1. Put beans in a large saucepan, add the water, bring to a boil over high heat, reduce temperature to medium low, cover and cook for 40 minutes.

2. In a food processor, mix garlic with salt, pepper, tomato and onion and pulse well.

3. Heat another saucepan with the oil over medium high heat, add tomato mix, stir and

cook for 5 minutes.

4. Add beans and their liquid, cumin and saffron, stir and cook for 10 more minutes.

5. Add more salt and pepper, stir, ladle into bowls and serve.

Nutrition Values:calories 213, fat 3, fiber 2, carbs 3, protein 8

34. Roasted Mushrooms with Quinoa

Preparation time: 10 minutes

Cooking time: 25 minutes

Servings:4

Ingredients:

- tablespoons olive oil
- Salt and black pepper to the taste
- 16 ounces mushrooms
- 1 cup quinoa
- 2 cups water
- ½ cup parmesan, grated
- ¼ cup parsley, chopped
- ¼ cup green onions, chopped
- 1 garlic clove, minced
- teaspoons lemon juice
- 2 tablespoons pepitas, toasted

Directions:

1. Arrange mushrooms on a lined baking sheet, add 1 tablespoon oil, salt and pepper and toss to coat.
2. Place in the oven at 425 degrees F and bake for 18 minutes.
3. Put water and quinoa in a pan, bring to a boil over medium high heat, reduce temperature, cook for 20 minutes, take off heat, cover, leave aside for 5 minutes and

fluff with a fork.

4. Add parmesan, parsley, salt, pepper, green onions and remaining oil and toss to coat.

5. Add lemon juice and stir again.

6. Divide quinoa on plates, add mushrooms on top, sprinkle pepitas all over and serve.

Nutrition Values:calories 132, fat 6, fiber 3, carbs 10, protein 7

35. Tasty Stuffed Peppers

Preparation time: 10 minutes

Cooking time: 20 minutes

Servings:4

Ingredients:

- 1 zucchini, chopped
- red peppers, cut in halves
- 2 tablespoons olive oil
- 17 ounces already cooked quinoa
- ounces feta cheese, crumbled
- Salt and black pepper to taste
- A handful parsley, finely chopped

Directions:

1. Place peppers on a lined baking sheet, drizzle 1 tablespoon oil, season with salt and pepper, place in the oven at 350 degrees F and cook for 15 minutes.
2. Heat a pan with remaining oil over medium heat, add zucchini, cook for 5 minutes, take off heat and mix with quinoa, salt, pepper, cheese and parsley and stir.
3. Take peppers out of oven, divide quinoa mix between them, place in the oven again and cook for 5 minutes more. Serve hot.

Nutrition Values:calories 245, fat 8, fiber 11, carbs 33, protein 11

36. Broad Bean Toast

Preparation time: 15 minutes

Cooking time: 5 minutes

Servings:2

Ingredients:

- 12 ounces broad bean
- ounces feta cheese, crumbled
- 1 tablespoon olive oil
- 2 tablespoons mint leaves, chopped
- Salt and black pepper to taste
- 2 ounces mixed salad leaves
- 10 cherry tomatoes, cut in halves
- 1 teaspoon lemon juice
- baguette slices

Directions:

Put some water in a saucepan, bring to a boil over medium high heat, add beans, cook for 4 minutes, drain and put into a bowl.

Add feta and mint, salt and pepper to taste and half of the oil and toss to coat.

In another bowl, mix tomatoes with salad leaves, some salt, pepper, lemon juice and the rest of the oil and toss to coat.

Divide this on serving plates, add toasted bread slices and top them with beans mix. Serve right away.

Nutrition Values:calories 354, fat 12, fiber 11, carbs 23, protein 20

37. Spinach with Chili

Preparation time: 10 minutes

Cooking time: 5 minutes

Servings:4

Ingredients:

- 1 tablespoon butter
- Zest from 1 lemon
- tablespoons bread crumbs
- 2 garlic cloves, minced
- 17 ounces spinach
- 1 red chili, chopped
- Salt and black pepper to taste

Directions:

Heat a pan with the butter over medium high heat, add breadcrumbs, garlic, chili and lemon zest, cook for 3 minutes, take off heat, transfer to a bowl and season with salt and pepper.

Heat the pan again over medium heat, add spinach, stir and cook for 2 minutes.

Divide spinach on plates, top with bread crumbs mix and serve.

Nutrition Values:calories 160, fat 7, fiber 3, carbs 20, protein 7

38. Spinach Dip

Preparation time: 15 minutes

Cooking time: 0 minutes

Servings:4

Ingredients:

- 1 bunch spinach, roughly chopped
- 1 scallion, sliced
- tablespoons mint, chopped
- ¾ cup sour cream
- Salt and black pepper to taste

Directions:

1. Put some water in a saucepan, bring to a boil over medium heat, add spinach, cook for 20 seconds, rinse and drain well, chop and put in a bowl.
2. Add sour cream, scallion, salt, pepper to taste, the mint, stir well, leave aside for 15 minutes and then serve.

Nutrition Values:calories 110, fat 1, fiber 1, carbs 1, protein 5

39. Artichoke Dip

Preparation time: 10 minutes

Cooking time: 30 minutes

Servings:10

Ingredients:

- ounces artichoke hearts
- ¾ cup basil, chopped
- ¾ cup green olive paste
- 1 cup parmesan cheese, grated
- ounces garlic and herb cheese

Directions:

1. In a food processor, mix artichokes with basil and pulse well.
2. Spread this into a baking dish, add olive paste, parmesan cheese, herbed cheese and stir.
3. Place in the oven at 375 degrees F and bake for 30 minutes. Serve warm.

Nutrition Values:calories 152, fat 2, fiber 3, carbs 3, protein 1

40. Simple Avocado Dip

Preparation time: 10 minutes

Cooking time: 0 minutes

Servings:8

Ingredients:

- ½ cup sour cream
- 1 chili pepper, chopped
- Salt and pepper to taste
- avocados, pitted, peeled and chopped
- 1 cup cilantro, chopped
- ¼ cup lemon juice
- Carrot sticks for serving

Directions:

1. Put avocados in a blender and pulse a few times.
2. Add sour cream and pulse again.
3. Add chili pepper, lemon juice, cilantro, salt and pepper to taste and pulse well again.
4. Transfer to a bowl and serve as a snack.

Nutrition Values:calories 112, fat 1, fiber 2, carbs 2, protein 4

41. Chive Dip

Preparation time: 10 minutes

Cooking time: 10 minutes

Servings:4

Ingredients:

- ounces goats cheese, soft
- ¾ cup sour cream
- 1 shallot, minced
- 1 tablespoon chives, chopped
- 1 tablespoon lemon juice
- Salt and black pepper to taste
- ½ pound potatoes, sliced
- ½ pound purple potatoes, sliced
- tablespoons extra virgin olive oil

Directions:

1. In a bowl, mix chives with sour cream, goat cheese, shallot, lemon juice, salt and pepper to taste and stir very well.
2. In another bowl, mix potato slices with salt and olive oil and toss to coat.
3. Heat up a grill pan over medium high heat, add potato slices, grill for 5 minutes on each side and transfer them to a bowl.
4. Serve your potato chips with the chive dip on the side.

Nutrition Values:calories 110, fat 2, fiber 2, carbs 2, protein 5

42. Chickpeas Appetizer

Preparation time: 10 minutes

Cooking time: 0 minutes

Servings:6

Ingredients:

- scallions, sliced

- 1 cup arugula, chopped

- 15 ounces canned chickpeas, chopped

- Salt and black pepper to taste

- 2 jarred red peppers, roasted and chopped

- 2 tablespoons olive oil

- 2 tablespoons lemon juice

Directions:

1. In a bowl, mix chickpeas with arugula, scallions, red peppers, salt, pepper, lemon juice and olive oil and stir very well.

2. Transfer to a bowl and serve.

Nutrition Values:calories 74, fat 2, fiber 2, carbs 6, protein 2

43. Cilantro Dip

Preparation time: 10 minutes

Cooking time: 0 minutes

Servings:6

Ingredients:

- ½ cup ginger, sliced
- 2 bunches cilantro, chopped
- tablespoons balsamic vinegar
- ½ cup olive oil
- 2 teaspoons sesame oil
- 2 tablespoons soy sauce

Directions:

1. In a blender mix cilantro with olive oil, ginger, vinegar, soy sauce and sesame oil and pulse very well. Transfer to a bowl and serve.

44. Chicken Salad with Toasted Pita Bread

Preparation time: 10 minutes

Cooking time: 5 minutes

Servings:4

Ingredients:

For the chicken:

- 1 tablespoon oregano, chopped

- garlic cloves, minced

- chicken breast halves, skinless and boneless

- 1 tablespoons lemon zest

- ¼ teaspoon water

- Salt and black pepper to taste

- 2 tablespoons parsley, chopped

- A drizzle of olive oil

- lemon wedges

For the salad:

- 2 pints cherry tomatoes cut in halves

- 1 small red onion, thinly sliced

- 1 cucumber, sliced

- 1 ½ tablespoons olive oil

- 1/3 cup black olives, pitted and cut in halves

- 1 cup tzatziki sauce

- Salt and black pepper to taste

- 1 teaspoon oregano, chopped

- pitas, toasted

Directions:

1. In a mortar, mix garlic with water, salt, pepper 1 teaspoon lemon zest and 1 tablespoon oregano and stir well.

2. Rub chicken pieces with this mix, drizzle them with some oil, put them on preheated grill pan over medium high heat, cook for 4 minutes, flip, cook for 1 minutes more, transfer to a plate, squeeze 2 lemon wedges over them, sprinkle parsley and leave aside for now.

3. In a salad bowl, mix tomatoes with olives, onion and cucumber.

4. Add salt, pepper, 1 ½ tablespoons oil and 1 teaspoon oregano, toss to coat and divide on serving plates.

5. Cut chicken breasts into strips and add on top of salad.

6. Drizzle tzatziki all over and serve with pitas and the remaining lemon wedges.

Nutrition Values:calories 400, fat 22, fiber 4, carbs 34, protein 34

45. Simple Spinach And Steak Salad

Preparation time: 5 hours

Cooking time: 10 minutes

Servings:4

Ingredients:

- 3 garlic cloves, minced
- ½ tablespoons olive oil
- 2 teaspoons red wine vinegar
- 1 tablespoons oregano, chopped
- Salt and black pepper to taste
- 2 tablespoons parsley, chopped
- 1 pound beef meat, sliced
- 1 tablespoon lemon juice
- 1 tablespoon capers, chopped
- 1 teaspoon thyme, chopped
- ounces feta cheese, cubed
- ¼ teaspoon red chili flakes
- 5 ounces baby spinach
- 2 cucumbers, thinly sliced
- 1 ½ cups cherry tomatoes cut in halves
- ½ cup kalamata olives, pitted and cut in halves

Directions:

1. In a bowl, mix 3 tablespoons oil with vinegar, oregano, garlic, salt and pepper and whisk.

2. Add beef meat, cover and keep in the fridge for 4 hours.

3. In another bowl, mix remaining oil with thyme, parsley, capers, lemon juice and chili flakes and whisk.

4. Add feta, toss to coat and leave aside for 1 hour.

5. Heat your kitchen grill pan over medium high heat, add beef pieces, grill for 8 minutes, turning every 2 minutes, transfer them to a cutting board, leave aside for cool down, thinly slice and season with salt and pepper to taste.

6. In a salad bowl, mix spinach with tomatoes, cucumber and olives.

7. Add feta and its marinade, salt and pepper to taste, toss to coat and divide on serving plates.

8. Top with steak pieces and serve.

9. Nutrition Values:calories 340, fat 32, fiber 4, carbs 11, protein 34

46. Grilled Potato Salad

Cooking time: 50 minutes

Servings:6

Ingredients:

- 4 sweet potatoes
- 3 tablespoons olive oil
- ¼ cup olive oil
- 1/3 cup orange juice
- 1 tablespoon orange juice
- 2 tablespoons pomegranate molasses
- ½ teaspoon sumac, ground
- 1 tablespoon red wine vinegar
- ½ teaspoon sugar
- Salt and black pepper to taste
- 1 tablespoon orange zest, grated
- 3 tablespoons honey
- 2 tablespoons mint, chopped
- 1/3 cup pistachios, chopped
- 1 cup Greek yogurt
- 1/3 cup pomegranate seeds

Directions:

1. Put potatoes on a lined baking sheet, place in the oven at 350 degrees F, bake for 40 minutes, leave them aside for 1 hour to cool down, peel them, cut into wedges and put on a cutting board.

2. In a bowl, mix ¼ cup oil with 1 tablespoon orange juice, sugar, vinegar, pomegranate molasses, sumac, salt and pepper and whisk.

3. In another bowl, mix the rest of the orange juice with orange zest, honey, salt, pepper and the remaining oil and whisk well again.

4. In a third bowl mix yogurt with some salt and pepper and with the mint and whisk.

5. Brush potato wedges with the honey mix, add some salt, place on your kitchen grill pan heated over medium high heat, cook for 3 minutes and transfer to serving plates.

6. Sprinkle pistachios, pomegranate seeds, drizzle the vinaigrette, and serve with the yogurt sauce on top.

Nutrition Values:calories 240, fat 14, fiber 3, carbs 32, protein 5

47. Cucumber Salad

Preparation time: 5 minutes

Cooking time: 0 minutes

Servings:4

Ingredients:

- 2 tablespoons olive oil
- 3 tablespoons red wine vinegar
- 1 teaspoon oregano, dried
- 3 cucumbers, peeled and thinly sliced
- Salt and black pepper to taste
- 1 small red onion, chopped
- ¼ cup feta cheese, crumbled
- 1 tablespoon dill, chopped

Directions:

1. In a bowl, mix oil with vinegar, oregano, salt and pepper and whisk well.
2. In a salad bowl, mix cucumber slices with onion, cheese and dill.
3. Add salad dressing, toss to coat and serve.

Nutrition Values:calories 53, fat 0.3, fiber 0.5, carbs 11, protein 1

48. Zesty Cabbage Salad

Preparation time: 10 minutes

Cooking time: 2 minutes

Servings:4

Ingredients:

- 1 teaspoon cumin, ground
- 1 small red onion, chopped
- 1 tablespoon olive oil
- 1 teaspoon coriander, ground
- 2 tablespoons lemon juice
- 2 teaspoons honey
- 1 tablespoon lemon zest, grated
- Salt and black pepper to taste
- 1 cup Greek yogurt
- 1 cabbage head, cut into halves and thinly sliced
- ½ cup mint, chopped
- 2 carrots, cut into thin strips
- ¼ cup pistachios, chopped

Directions:

1. Put the onion in a bowl, add water to cover, leave aside for 20 minutes, drain and put in a bowl. Heat a pan over medium high heat, add oil cumin and coriander, stir, cook for 2 minutes, take off heat and leave aside to cool down.

2. Add salt, pepper, lemon juice, lemon zest, honey and yogurt and stir well.

3. In a salad bowl, mix cabbage with onion, mint and carrots.

4. Add salad dressing, sprinkle pistachios, toss to coat and leave aside for 10 minutes before serving.

5. Add more salt and pepper to taste and serve.

Nutrition Values:calories 139, fat 5, fiber 5, carbs 13, protein 5

49. Scampi Provencale - Shrimp Prawn Recipe

Ingredients:

- Olive oil (for frying)

- Finely chopped, peeled medium onion- 1

- Crushed and peeled garlic cloves – 3

- Olive oil – 2 tbsp

- Tomato purée – 1tsp

- White wine – 50ml (a splash)

- Roughly chopped tomatoes – 10 or can of chopped tomatoes – 400g

- Fresh black pepper and salt

- Chopped parsley – a handful

- Cornstarchcornflour – ½ (if necessary slacked with water a little)

Directions:

1. Prepare the sauce firstly by having the garlic and onion fried inside a frying pan that is non-sticky with olive oil for some minutes without giving it color

2. Have the tomato purée stirred in, zest, lemon juice, and white wine. Allow it simmer for one minute

3. Add your tomatoes, have it seasoned and let it simmer for 5 to 6 minutes till the tomatoes are beginning to open up

4. Have the prawns shrimps added and allow it to simmer till it has turned to pink. This

takes about 3 to 4 minutes. Be careful about having it overcooked

5. If many juices come out from the scampi shrimp while cooking, it might be necessary to have the sauce thickened by using the cornflour mixture. Just have it stirred in and let it simmer

6. Have the chopped parsley stirred in and check your seasoning

7. Have it stirred immediately with vegetables or rice.

50. The Lubina a la sal – Sea Bass

Ingredients:

- Cleaned whole sea bass – 2 (¼lb or 550g)

- Coarse sea salt – 4 (½lb or 2k)

- Crushed garlic clove – 1

- Extra virgin olive oil – 4tbls.

- Fresh lemon juice – 2tbls.

- Salt – 1 leveled tsp.

- Honey – 2tsps.

- Dried dill – 1 heaped tsp.

- Aromatic chili oil – 1 Tsp.

Directions:

1. Firstly, have a big earthenware dish laid (it should be big enough to have the fish in without it touching the sides) along with a ½ inch of salt

2. Take the dish and lay it on the salt

3. Put the remaining salt on top of it

4. Have it patted down and have little water sprinkled on top of it to keep it moist

5. Have the earthenware placed inside an oven that is preheated to 400oF or 200oC for about 30 minutes

6. Have your sauce prepared- have all the Ingredients: put inside a glass bowl except the oil

7. Have the oil whisked in a tablespoon one at a time using a hand whisk

8. Have the fish eaten out of the oven, turn it down to low and put in the dinner plates to make it warm

9. The salt would have turned into a crust that is hard, so have it broken with a mallet gently and remove it from the fish

10. The skin would come off easily, and you can be able to have the fillets removed and have them arranged on the dinner plates

11. You can have the sauce sprinkled and begin to eat

12. If it's the traditional method you prefer- make use of a pinch of salt and have the lemon juice squeezed.

CPSIA information can be obtained
at www.ICGtesting.com
Printed in the USA
BVHW011948161121
621792BV00019B/192

9 781801 789936